INTERMITTENT FASTING STRUCTURES

By Sean McDowell

LEGAL DISCLAIMER:

The Publisher has strived to be as accurate and complete as possible in the creation of this report, even though he does not warrant or represent at any time that the contents within are accurate due to the rapidly changing nature of the Internet.

Any viewed slights of specific persons, individuals, or companies are unintended. The purpose of this book is to educate, and there are no guarantees of income, sales or results implied. The publisher/author/reseller can, for that reason, not be held accountable for any bad results you may attain when implementing the methods or when following any standards set out for you in this book.

The author and publisher shall have neither liability nor responsibility to any person or entity concerning any loss or damage caused or alleged to be caused directly or indirectly by this book

INTRODUCTION

It's nearly difficult to hide from the news and discussion about the obesity epidemic that's taking both lives and shattering the lifestyle world large. It remains in the papers, on tv, and being blogged about on the internet almost constantly.

If that's inadequate, unless you're blind it's tough to stroll the streets of any big city or village and not see the completion item of this epidemic first hand. The tough ruthless fact is that individuals are getting fatter and fatter and this is a real health crisis that only a fool might neglect.

There's a lot of factors for this here that are just the most blindingly evident ...

Many Individuals Eat Method too Much Way frequently.

It's a hard truth that can't be gotten away. The body wasn't developed by nature to eat as much and as typically as most people do. This packs on the sagging pounds as our bodies, which are machines that were developed for survival in not so terrific circumstances are pampered and overfed in a cushy and soft environment. Eliminate a bit of appetite from our lives and we will load on fat and pack it on at warp speed.

A Widespread Avoidance of Exercise.

After eating way too much the next big problem is under-exercising. Having less physical tasks in addition to social lives that revolve around the digital rather than the physical once again takes our bodies away from what they were developed for: running, lifting, searching, and playing. The less muscle we bring the lower our metabolic process which means a lot more fat is packed on. Do you see a pattern developing?

Absence of Quality Sleep.

The first 2 obesity contractors add to the 3rd. Poor diet and lack of exercise use the fast lane to broken sleep patterns which have been shown in more studies than can be counted to also damage metabolism and pack on fat. Sleepless nights tossing and turning rapidly equal an unsightly spare tire of fat around the waist.

Medicine and Drugs

Coming along with our progressively over-medicated society are the side effects of all these medications, which typically consist of weight gain and sleepiness. Cultures who approach health more naturally and holistically have largely prevented this problem and have been likewise able to prevent the weight problems associated with health issues that come along with it. Our societies for the most part haven't figured this out yet.

These are just a few of the many factors the obesity afflict is spreading out in such a quick and deadly manner. There's plenty more, trust me.

The concern stands - what can we do about it? How can we turn the tide against obesity? The response is, naturally, diet plan and exercise. There are lots of varied ideas about both, some great and a few bad. This guide provides what I feel may be the ideal option for a huge majority of individuals who struggle with putting on fat.

It's relatively simple and packed with power, in line with both nature and common sense. Most significantly it works and works almost like magic. It's called the Feast and Famine Diet and it can change your life for the better. After reading this you will be armed with all you need to know about Feast and Famine to make it work and get the lean and healthy body of your dreams.

Prepare this is going to be a blast!

CHAPTER 1

<u>WHAT IS THE FEAST AND FAMINE DIET?</u>

The Feast and Famine Diet might be brand-new in name, however, in practice has been with us for quite a long time. It's the current tweak on a location of diet programs and ideas less catching described as Intermittent Fasting. Intermittent Fasting is the rage in health, fitness, and weight reduction circles with its concepts making it to publication and wide practice. It's popular since it works!

Here are the important directing principles of Feast and Famine, what offers the diet its power. Attempt not to stray too far from this foundation if you expect to reap the full rewards of Feast and Famine ...

Pick Your Fasting Schedule

There are 2 methods usually. The first is rotating Feast days with Famine days, which is personally the technique I have seen produce the very best weight-loss outcomes. The second variant and this is what you will see in periodic fasting diets like the 5:2 Diet is to consume normally five days and quick 2. Our Guide's details work well with both approaches, although once again I choose the very first for best long-term results in addition to ease of use and probability of having the ability to stick to Feast and Famine.

Feasting Standards

There are not many. I suggest broadly not eating anything that's unhealthy food or packed with empty calories particularly if you are looking to burn off a great deal of weight. This will also protect your overall health, which is necessary, isn't it?

Make sure you get in your fruit and vegetables but don't hesitate to indulge without binge consuming. The truth you have more food flexibility a minimum of half the time will make your Famine days a lot easier to handle psychology.

And prospering on any diet, Feast and Famine consisted of, is 90% a psychological game. In this psychological dieting video game, no diet stacks the deck more in your favor than Feast and Famine.

Famine Guidelines

For those requiring to drop major pounds, 500 calories a day on Famine days is a good beginning point. This can be adjusted as required once your weight reduction goals are satisfied. A Lot Of Feast and Famine enthusiasts like to remain around this area to continue to both reap the health advantages of fasting and to likewise be able to preserve their Feasting liberty on their Feast days.

Stay Hydrated. Fasting specialist or if you have never fasted in any kind before alike, I can not worry enough about the importance of remaining hydrated. When your body detoxes on your Famine days and starts to leave some of the junk you have developed, it will go much smoother if you are consuming the correct amount of water.

Neglect this advice and you might simply experience some stomach discomforts, in addition to the lethargy and weakness that always comes with dehydration no matter your diet strategy. One of the best strengths of intermittent fasting and the Feast and Famine Diet is its simpleness. No diet logs, carb manipulation schemes, and other problems. It works much more dramatically than diets that you need a flow diagram to follow too.

If you can't stay with Feast and Famine it has absolutely nothing to do with being confused, however with a lack of willpower, self-discipline, and most of all desire. I think you have those covered, do not you?

CHAPTER 2

THE BEGINNING OF THE FEAST & FAMINE DIET

Every good concept got its start somewhere. The every other day Feast and Famine Diet has had its method paved for it by earlier intermittent fasting procedures, some a big impact and others not so much, but who still are worthy of credit for being forward thinkers.

Let's take a look at the history of diets that have come before Feast and Famine and see what we can gain from them. Knowledge is power after all. We have already seen in the mirror and felt in our bodies - that Feast and Famine work big time, we have these speed setters to thank for their experiments and innovations!

First The Warrior.

Make no mistake, Ori Hofmekler is certainly a unique guy. Artist, author, and ex-special forces soldier who ran a brief-lived fitness publication that was released by a popular Male's publication business. During his time as editorial director, he was exposed to the typically conflicting concepts of a who's who of dieting masters of the time, which landed him a fascination with getting to the reality about weight loss.

A couple of years later came the Warrior Diet book which promotes a 16 hour daily quick followed by an 8-hour consuming period. General agreement was that it worked, however, most people feel the Warrior Diet is tough to keep, far more so than every other day fasting ala Feast and Famine. In either case, Ori gets credit for the modern birth of intermittent fasting and has worked as a fantastic influence on a lot of everybody's ideas who are dealing with these techniques.

Eat Stop Eat.

Eat Stop Eat has been an intermittent fasting dieting technique promoted most just recently by Brad Pillon. Brad pushes the concept of a couple of, absolutely no calorie days a week, the rest of the days eating generally. Once again it works and close to what we recommend, however, our experience has shown decreasing to 500 calories every other day is much more efficient and manageable than a couple of days of no calories at all. Not many seem to be able to stick with Eat Stop Eat for long in our experience.

The 5:2 Diet.

This is the diet strategy most closely related to Feast and Famine and also closest to us on the timeline. It's extremely popular in Europe and is gaining ground in places like Hollywood in the U.S.A.. 5 days of typical eating followed by two days of lowered calories. Very effective and all our ideas here work well with the 5:2 Diet. Our opinion holds every other day Feast and Famine is a much better fat burner without added mental tolls. Follow this Guide's advice and I believe you will concur!

That's the current history of intermittent fasting leading us to where we are today. Feast and Famine are today and I believe it will proudly stand the test of time. It torches fat, is simple to follow, requires no added expenditures in its purest kind, and promotes overall vibrant health.

What exists not to like about Feast and Famine?
It's best for the health enthusiast who wishes to get lean and look excellent.

CHAPTER 3

THE BENEFITS OF THE FEAST & FAMINE DIET

The Feast and Famine Diet brings a load of advantages some more apparent than others. Are you ready to take a look? I believe you'll find them truly exciting. If significantly lowering fat while likewise indulging in these health advantages does not interest somebody looking to change their body for the better I'm unsure what will!

Rapidly Cut Body Fat Safely

This is why many people will explore the Feast and Famine method to diet. You can anticipate seeing the fat melt off as long as you take your Famine Day seriously. Eat too much on those days and you are undoubtedly missing the point. We understand this works, we have seen it, and now even much better news - science backs it up!

A recent University of Illinois research study has shown in those following alternate-day lowered calorie strategies (in line with our Guide's suggestions) lost significantly more fat than those consuming generally and following the very same exercise procedures. It's a plus to be on the right side of science when, sadly, they most often track far behind the true health and diet vanguard!

Easy To Follow And Manage

The next groundbreaking advantage of Feast and Famine is how easy it is to follow and manage. I have discussed this already, however it truly bears duplicating. Anybody who has counted carbohydrates on a ketogenic diet like Atkins or the many others I make sure will rapidly concur! Once you find out in your head what your 500 or 600 calories on famine days look like you are set. No calculators or complications, period.

Improved Mental Function

Yes, we presumed it, however, science has backed us up once again. Lowered weekly calories (which is what you get with the Feast and Famine Diet) leads to increased focus, better memory, and other improved cognitive function according to Mark Mattson's research for the Lancet. These effects might even carry over into the fight versus Alzheimer's disease and other comparable big health issues which Mattson is exploring even more.

Improve Insulin Levels

One of the reasons lots of people load on and discover it so hard to lose body fat is theirs out-of-whack insulin levels. The Feast and Famine technique enhances insulin levels for healthy weight loss, which simply adds to the amount of fat currently being cut from the calorie reduction and heightened metabolic process we've currently discussed.

Maximizes Time On Famine Days

One of the surprising advantages of this technique is the newfound time you discover available on Famine Day. Little meals and no constant snacking or grazing frees up a shocking amount of time and energy that can be used positively in other places. I have discovered, and others have verified this, that some of our most imaginative and efficient days end up again and again to be famine days! Far from not having energy, you end up filled with it!

The Feast and Famine Diet method is loaded with advantages, physical, psychological, and even social. It's hard to even think about anything, however a little disadvantage or 2 and then just for those who are doing not have in the desire to "get lean" department. This is genuinely a method that changes lives for the best.

CHAPTER 4
<u>GETTING YOURSELF READY TO BEGIN</u>

Any diet requires a little bit of preparation, in the beginning, Feast and Famine is certainly not an exception. I will state it requires much less preparation by the nature of Feast and Famine than any other diet I can consider and you will not have to jump many difficulties, do any real pricey shopping, or experience any of the other more standard diet head pains.

Here are some ideas to obtain ready to get the most out of our plan ...

Read And Understand This Guide

It's quite short so why not even read it twice. I have done my best to keep it fluff-free and all the details and suggestions will make your journey at intermittent fasting Feast and Famine design much, a lot easier. If you like to read take a look at a few of the books in our history chapter and you may find some other ideas you want to integrate after you've done straight Feast and Famine for a bit.

If Possible In The Beginning Food Store More Frequently

Here's a technique I utilized in the beginning days of my intermittent fasting experiments and I have recommended it to a lot of my friends and clients who have provided it high praise too. Only keep enough food on hand for the day's needs. On Feasting days you will have the pleasure of picking out some brand-new reward to enjoy and on Famine days you won't be as lured to cheat as you would be if the refrigerator is loaded with snacks. Now if you live rurally, or have a big family this might be less practical, however, if you can do it I ensure it will give you a big advantage over those who ignore this suggestion.

If You Skip A Day Just Get Right Back On Schedule

This diet is about liberty and abundance, not a constraint. If you have a family event, a date, or even a small slip up on a Famine day just solve back in action the next day and lower your calories. No master dietary equations are fouled or other rubbish. Now do not make practice of this or you may end up seeing less than optimal results, once in a while is completely great. This automatic freedom is constructed into the Feast and Famine program making it not a diet you can "fail" at if you stumble while getting into the groove, or any other time truly!

Throw away Your Previous Diet Experiences

Feast and Famine requires an entirely new view of dieting, so in all likelihood, your previous dieting experiences favorable and particularly unfavorable don't offer a great deal of relevance. I'd recommend you submit them away and don't let them influence what you are doing here and now. This mindset, not only in dieting and fitness but also in other areas of life can break chains and open doors. See what you believe.

Are you feeling more all set to begin? You ought to be because there's a bright, healthy, and pleased brand-new you waiting at the end of the Feast and Famine road. And it's a roadway not particularly long in many cases and even exceptionally hard. You have taken the first step by reading this Guide, do not reverse now!

CHAPTER 5

<u>COMMON BEGINNER MISTAKES</u>

Now even if the Feast and Famine Diet is easy to understand and simple to apply to your way of life does not suggest it's easy for all to practice or it's impossible to make errors. Some errors with intermittent fasting are relatively common among beginners, let's go over them and see if you can't avoid these mistakes before you make them instead of after. A few of these I even found out the hard way!

Pigging Out on Excessive on Junk Food

Let's be serious for a second on the subject of getting lean and healthy. While we are permitted and encouraged to eat loosely and enjoyably on Feast days this doesn't suggest we have a license to eat completely like a glutton.

So if you are not losing weight the way you want to be and are consuming unlimited chips, ice cream, and candy on your Feast days tighten up your diet and consume healthier. You should be striving to enhance your health anyhow, shouldn't you?

Being Scared to Death of Appetite

No one has ever starved to death consuming 500 calories or less every other day. Nor have they damaged their body in any way. So if you are experiencing terrific tension and pain over being hungry every other day, it's time to get more control over your mind. This is done by establishing your willpower doing things like following this diet even when you would rather not be, focusing on your preferred outcome. Be tough and be rewarded.

Eating Too Much On Famine Days

Let's not play games, 500 calories or fewer methods 500 calories or less. If you are eating tidy on your Feast days and still not dropping weight it likely methods you are consuming too much on Famine days. Reduce what you are eating and if you should inspect the calorie counts to make certain you are at 500 calories or under.

Reducing Your Level of Activity

It's tempting for some to decrease their activities on Famine Day. Don't fall under this. In fact, with a little Feast and Famine experience under your belt, you will understand Famine days free up more energy and you ought to strive to be much more active. Doing more is almost always much better than doing nothing as long as you can do it safely.

Putting Yourself Unnecessarily Around Individuals Who Don't Respect Your Diet Efforts.

Apart from buddies and households who it would be hard to prevent, it's a downer to be around people who try to talk adversely about or discourage you from fulfilling your Feast and Famine goals. Again dieting is 90% mental so don't let other people mess with your mental video game. It's bothersome, defeatist, and unneeded!

These common beginner mistakes are all easy to avoid and if you stumble it's okay simply keep going. The Feast and Famine Diet has been created to be both reliable, open, and easy to use. A little bit of self-reflection and you are quickly back on course and taking the body and life of your dreams!

CHAPTER 6

A SAMPLE FEAST DAY

The Feast and Famine Feast Day! Now comes the enjoyable part, my friends! Let's dig deep into a sample Feast day while we are following the Feast and Famine Diet. This is drawn from my lifestyle and from an amount of time when I was regularly reducing weight as quickly as I ever had each week without fail. My metabolic process has never been superhuman either, so felt confident if this has worked for me it's very, likely to work for you too (with part sizes adjusted if you are female, naturally.).

Read on and enjoy. I hope it gets you filled with interest! You will notice I'm not consisting of calories, because who counts calories on a Feast day?! I sure don't and you shouldn't either.

Breakfast.

Breakfast is concerned by numerous nutrition professionals as being the most essential meal of the day. It's also a meal I've neglected most of my life due to the dangers of delighting in sleeping in. Intermittent fasting has cleared that up - after a 500 calorie day I can't wait to truly eat a significant breakfast! I need to say I feel much more all set for action after a full force breakfast.

4 Eggs Scrambled. I select to opt for whole eggs for hormonal optimization's sake, however typically blend the ways the eggs are prepared.
Fresh Tomato, Onion, and Jalapeno Salsa. Extra hot and used as a dressing on top of my eggs.
4 pieces of Turkey Bacon. I will consume other designs of bacon when turkey bacon isn't readily available.

4oz of Steak Sauteed in a Frying Pan. I just add this when I want to indulge or if I feel like I require the extra protein for bodybuilding purposes.
8oz Milk. Whole milk is also fantastic for men looking to naturally boost their hormone benefits.

Snack.
A couple of hands filled with Organic Almonds.

Small Spinach Salad. I don't use dressing beyond olive oil and garlic and sometimes toss in some tomatoes, onion, and cucumber depending on what's on hand.

Lunch.

Medium Baked Potato. I dress the potato with a little butter and garlic.
2 6oz Grilled Chicken Breasts. Sometimes plain or sometimes with salsa on top if I have additional from breakfast.

Snack.
More Almonds!

Dinner.

10oz Grilled Lean Steak. Plain beyond salt and pepper.
Little side salad or spinach salad.
Side Portion of White or Wild Rice.
As much **Green Tea** as I wish to consume sweetened with pure stevia.
Periodically a desert of organic sorbet, a little addiction of mine!

Snack.

My after-dinner snack is quite wide open within reason.
If I eat chips I ensure to not overdo it.

Vanilla Whey Protein shakes made with half whole milk and half almond milk. I consume this right before bed.

This is just a sample Feast and Famine Feast day, but it should provide you a terrific concept of what's possible when we consume smartly and perfectly. The genuine eye-opener is when you consume like this half the time and still see the fat melting away. That's when you will end up being a full force Feast and Famine true believer!

CHAPTER 7

A SAMPLE FAMINE DAY

Now after seeing a sample Feast and Famine Feast day it's time for a sample of the other side - the all-important Famine day where we will quickly consuming greatly reduced calories activating our metabolic process, our "skinny gene" and setting ourselves up for both body improvement and all the other health benefits we have already discussed. This is once again, from my own experience and the everyday calorie total is focused on the magic number of 500 calories. I believe you will discover this a manageable day that will hardly leave you suffering.

Pre-Breakfast

16oz Sparkling water immediately upon wakening.
A cup of Fresh Coffee, no milk or cream sweetened with stevia. 0 calories.

Breakfast

The 2nd cup of Fresh Coffee, no milk or cream sweetened with stevia. 0 calories.
8oz Spring Water.

Now, this does not look like much of a breakfast, but I prefer to sleep in a bit and save my calories for lunch and dinner. This is my option and you might select to disperse your calories differently if you are more of a morning person!

Snack
8oz Green Tea sweetened with stevia. 0 calories.
12oz Sparkling water.

Lunch

Lastly, time to get in some food, paying unique objective NOT to overdo
it. This is the meal when many feel most lured, considering that while
consuming a little dinner you know a big breakfast is showing up
reasonably quickly. Do not give up!

2 medium tough boiled eggs. Once again I like to make sure I consume
entire eggs every day to optimize my hormone optimization strategy. You
have the choice of egg whites, egg beaters, and so on. 175 Calories.
Two pieces Whole Wheat Toast. Sometimes I eat the eggs on the toast
and in some cases as a side depending on the state of mind. 115 Calories.
A cup of Fresh Coffee, no milk or cream sweetened with stevia. 0
calories.
8oz spring water.

Overall Lunch calories: 290 offer or take.

Snack
8oz Green Tea sweetened with stevia. 0 calories. Yes, I do love caffeine
on Famine day in case you were questioning. It serves to boost energy,
raise metabolic processes, and even acts as a moderate cravings
suppressant.
12oz Springwater.

Dinner

Half a cup (after prepared) Spaghetti with a small amount of low
fat/low-calorie butter, salt, pepper, and garlic. 150 calories.
One-piece whole wheat toast. 55 calories.
12oz Spring Water.

Total calorie intake for the day roughly 495 calories. This puts us right where we are wishing to be on a Famine day. I repeat these meals often considering that they are decision complimentary and basic to prepare. They can likewise quickly be ordered in all but the most unskilled of dining establishments!

One last bit of recommendations - take a half-hour on Sunday and figure out your five hundred calories and listed below meals for the week rather than just attempting to wing it and think how many calories you are consuming on Famine days on the fly.

This will end up equating to much more weight loss over the long term and also conserve you a couple of headaches and a bit of possible confusion too. When in doubt repeat meals! Do not fret about getting bored a Feast day is less than 24 hours away!

CHAPTER 8

<u>SHOPPING GUIDELINES</u>

Now that we ideally have agreed that the Feast and Famine Diet is more than do-able after looking at a sample Feast day and a sample Famine day I thought I'd share with you a few more intermittent fasting insider's tricks.

The art of shopping while following Feast and Famine. Although everyone develops our design of consuming while on the diet which finest matches our requirements I have found having an experienced veteran's wish list can offer some practical standards. So are you all set to go shopping Feast and Famine style? Let's do it!

Here's what we are packing our shopping cart with ...

Non-hormonal Chicken Breasts. I'm a bit of a chicken addict and don't think I might live without it. I eat chicken at least once a day on Feast days, often twice. I think about chicken as a sort of "neutral" protein that can be prepared in numerous ways it's a good idea to fall for.

Make sure the fat is cut off!

Non-hormonal Grass Fed Lean Beef. Another Feast day favorite, particularly when I'm striking it more heavily in the fitness center. When you are aiming to place on muscle while cutting fat on Feast and Famine go for around 1 gram of protein for every single pound you weigh.

Eggs. As you have seen eggs are on the meal agenda frequently for both Feast and Famine days. Do not avoid them, unless you are among the few who can't stand the thought of them!

A variety of Pasta.

Organic Spinach

Organic Leaf Lettuce. I must add natural produce is not a must, however, I attempt to stick with it when I can.

Tomatoes.

Onions.

Miso soup. Miso soup is terrific for a change of rate on Famine days and has been displayed in research study to have all sorts of regenerative and health-enhancing qualities. Plus it tastes great too!

Green Tea. Essential. Green Tea is great for an extra fat loss increase, is low-cost, and calorie complimentary.

Coffee.

Spring Water.

Whey Protein. I have attempted to prevent any supplement suggestions as the Feast and Famine Diet works terrific without them, but a great protein shake is the one exception. Keep your protein levels high and you will have no concerns at all about losing muscle while cutting body fat.

Stevia. A 100% natural and calorie-free sweetener that will make you forget sugar ever even existed. A true gift from above.

Almonds. A go-to snack.

Now a look at this list reveals that preventing overly processed and unhealthy food isn't a bad idea and you can still truly Feast without it. That way if you go a bit crazy at a pal's or eating out sometimes your body won't even see it. Buying too many terrible food choices probably sends the wrong message to your subconscious and may establish many for binge eating and failure. Some intermittent fasting experts disagree, however, this is what my own experience has exposed.

After you move beyond the novice phase feel free to experiment!

CHAPTER 9

INCORPORATING THE FEAST & FAMINE DIET INTO YOUR LIFESTYLE LONGTERM

The only method to reduce weight and keep it off is to make the psychological switch from believing in terms of short-term dieting to the more dynamic perspective of making enduring healthy way of life choices. Feast and Famine is the ideal tool to help you make that change. In fact, after studying and experimenting with every significant diet of the last years, I can honestly state none, in my opinion, are much better suited for a long-term lifestyle choice than intermittent fasting and Feast and Famine.

It's simple to handle, low-cost to follow, fairly enjoyable and pleasurable, and extremely, very effective.
This covers nearly every category of a dream long-term consuming strategy checklist I can think of! Here are some suggestions in integrating Feast and Famine into your lifestyle long term ...

Celebrate Your Successes With Feast And Famine.

Believing positive and picking to concentrate on the favorable changes you have made while intermittent fasting will go a long way in solidifying it as a part of your lasting way of life. Try your finest to not dwell on any poor weeks or bumps in the road you may experience. This will pay off huge dividends both in weight reduction and in life. Once again 90% of the video game is psychological, let's not forget.

Recruit Those Closest To You To Lend A Hand

Making your better half friends and household familiar with how Feast and Famine work and letting them know you might use their assistance encouraging you to be disciplined on Famine days will assist this healthy lifestyle cement itself in place. Some might even pick to take up the Feast and Famine flag themselves when they see how excellent you look and feel. That's when you understand you are really onto something!

Take A Week Off Every Few Months

Everyone requires a trip periodically. This will avoid burnout and offer yourself a great pat on the back after months of discipline. If you can time your vacation from Feast and Famine with a genuine holiday from work or school even much better! I've found a week off assists recharge enthusiasm's batteries and allows me to plunge back into the Feast and Famine way of life full blast.

Keep Expanding Your Knowledge Of Intermittent Fasting

The last method to ensure you stick to Feast and Famine as a way of life option is to keep your brain participated in discovering new knowledge about intermittent fasting in all its types. Join some online forums, follow the news and the blogs and if you go to a health club make good friends with others living in this manner of life. This will continually validate what you are doing is both a healthy and a good option. It's always an excellent idea to have as huge an assistance circle as possible.

Even if you use up Feast and Famine to lose some weight quickly preparing to go back to your old methods of consuming, let me warn you, you might effectively wind up connected and sticking around for the duration. The good news is your body will be much healthier and look much better for your efforts. Breaking from the norm into a lifestyle that gets the most out of mind and body is an invaluable advantage. Embrace it!

CONCLUSION

TIPS TO BEGIN YOUR DIET JOURNEY TODAY

Thanks for making the effort to read our Guide and I hope you have discovered it practical and eye-opening. I do not doubt if you toss your focus into the Feast and Famine Diet you will achieve your weight loss goals and far more.

That stated when do you plan to start? If you just hesitated you might be experiencing the best opponent of attaining the body of your imagine them all - the evil called procrastination. Before I leave let me show you some suggestions that can help you kill that monster and begin your own improvement story today!

Just Do It

The Feast and Famine Diet requires no unique food, no supplements, and no info, actually, beyond this Guide to work and work well. So what are you waiting for? Start Feast and Famine today. The only thing stopping you is your inertia. Eliminate any ideas of tomorrow or next week. Once again make a decision and begin NOW.

Expose Your Excuses

Do you have repeating excuses why you can't begin intermittent fasting today? State these reasons aloud so you can hear how extremely self-defeating they are. If you are still in doubt write them down and burn them as you complimentary yourself from limiting beliefs.

Take a look at Yourself Naked In The Mirror.

If you are fat the mirror and an absence of clothes will not lie. Remind yourself your body won't change into something more pleasing until you first decide to change it and then 2nd progress with action in support of that decision. That action is to sensibly adopt the Feast and Famine Diet. If not you will likely look the same, if not even worse than you carried out in the mirror in the days, weeks, months, and years to come. This may sound severe, but an extreme fact is better than an enjoyable fallacy.

Quit Time Wasters.

Do you need so many social networks, television, or playing computer games when your body isn't where you desire it to be? Are you putting the easy and distracting before the essential and important? If so why? Break the hypnotic trance, stopped the time-wasters, and build the brand-new you NOW!

Write Your Goals Down As Clearly And Detailed As Possible.

There's a particular magic about the written word, specifically when it concerns setting and attaining goals. This magic is much more noticeable when the written words are your own. Jot down your goals big and small, read them, and accept Feast and Famine as a means to bring you in the instructions you require to be headed. There isn't a successful coach or sports psychologist alive who would argue against that advice! You shouldn't either.

Are you psyched about progressing with Feast and Famine? I understood you would be. This could be a day you review decades from now and state "that's where I dedicated to severe life-enhancing change!" The important things provided by this lifestyle are just that serious. I'd enjoy hearing your success story so please remain strong and in touch!